MW01298025

Disclaimer

This book contains content generated by us. The content in this book is provided for general information only. It is not intended to amount to advice on which you should rely. In particular, this information is not a substitute for professional medical care by a qualified doctor or other healthcare professional. If you are not a healthcare professional then you should ALWAYS check with your doctor if you have any concerns about your condition or treatment and before taking, or refraining from, any action on the basis of the content on our book. If you are a healthcare professional then this information (including any professional reference material) is intended to support, not replace, your own knowledge, experience and judgement.

Copyright

Copyright 2015 - All rights reserved.

This document is geared towards providing exact and reliable information in regards to the topic and issue covered. The publication is sold with the idea that the publisher is not required to render accounting, officially permitted, or otherwise, qualified services. If advice is necessary, legal or professional, a practiced individual in the profession should be ordered.

In no way is it legal to reproduce, duplicate, or transmit any part of this document in electronic means or in a printed format. Recording of this publication is strictly prohibited and any storage of this document is not allowed unless with written permission from the publisher. All rights reserved.

Table of Contents

Introduction

A busy and tiring lifestyle can definitely cause negative effects on a person's health and well-being. Combined with stressful work schedules, hectic days and poor eating habits, it would not be surprising that a lot of people have been suffering from several health-related problems such as body pains, weight gain, diabetes, hypertension and increase in cholesterol levels.

Have you ever experienced waking up in the morning feeling sluggish, tired and heavy? If you have, then it may be time for you to reflect on your daily activities and, of course, on your eating habits and the food that you eat. And with all the junk food and fast food meals that we can get, the increase in the number of people experiencing these health and behavior related problems is definitely expected.

Of course you can cut back on your food in Use and hit the gym as often as you can, but again, once your schedule gets in the way, then you will be back to your poor, old habits. Such pattern can be seen not just on a selected few, but on millions and millions of people, including you and me.

Yes! This so-called "solution" has been my demise — having tried and failed at this for so many times; you can imagine how much my health and even my attitude towards getting fit and healthy have deteriorated. And the fact that I am overworked and too busy to spend time preparing and following a diet plan, it wasn't surprising that I have reached the point where I wanted to throw in the towel and just go with the flow.

And just before I declared and admitted defeat, I was introduced to juicing and vitamin water! And believe it when I say that vitamin water has changed my eating habits, improved my health and my attitude towards life, in general.

You might be a bit of a skeptic about this, but this book will surely provide you with really important yet simple information about:

- What vitamin water is
- The benefits of vitamin water
- Recipes that you can try and
- How you can keep up with this improved way of drinking water.

This book is not just about instructions and tips; it also includes the personal aspect of things. Read on and discover that there is an easier and better way to achieving the best and the healthiest version of you — ever!

Chapter One

What is Vitamin Miracle Water?

Water has been part of every living creature's life. Which means that without it, there would not be anything on earth. Its nurturing properties are very important when it comes to rehydrating the body, as well as the distribution of nutrients that our bodies need to survive and stay healthy.

It has been determined that for the body to continue functioning properly, a person should drink at least 8 glasses of water every single day. But what if you are not a water drinker like me? How will you be able to keep yourself hydrated and completely energized? Well if you answered that you could always Use vitamin supplements and drink fruit juices that you can buy from the groceries, then you can join the thousands, if not, millions of people who share the same mindset.

And while fruit juices and other artificial sports drinks which promise to hydrate the body can work most of the time, you cannot deny the fact that these have preservatives that can or may do your body more harm than good — no matter how much they try to convince you that these are all made from natural ingredients. So as a really effective alternative, why don't you try vitamin infused water instead?

What is Fruit Water?

Vitamin water, not to be confused with juicing — the name actually speaks for itself, being loaded with vitamins and minerals in their most natural form. It is infused with different kinds of fresh fruits, vegetables, and herbs without the presence of artificial sugar or sweeteners and flavorings.

This can be considered as a more flavorful alternative to your usual bottled water and of course, a healthier alternative to your canned juices, fizzy drinks, sodas, sports drinks and those vitamin infused waters which are commercially produced.

So if you are not fond of plain tasting drinks but also do not like to fill yourself with unhealthy beverages, then vitamin water is definitely something that you can use to properly hydrate yourself

Chapter Two

Why Homemade Vitamin Water Is Superior

Before learning about the different benefits of making your very own vitamin water, it is also important to make sure that you are thinking about juicing when you hear vitamin water.

While juicing may require you to process and breakdown fruits and vegetables to get their juices in the process of juicing, vitamin water will not ask you to bring out your juicer or machine to get your bottles of infused water ready.

Aside from not using a machine to create vitamin loaded drinking water, there are more reasons for choosing this option.

Reasons for Going for Homemade Vitamin Water

Of course you have the choice of buying those bottled vitamin water brands available at your local groceries and even health food stores, but if you are a purist and you really want to give more weight to your belief of feeding your body with all natural types of food, then you should definitely try out making your very own vitamin water at home.

Not only will you know what you are putting in your body, you will also have the chance to cater to your taste all the more. You will be encouraged to get creative to put different flavors together. At the same time, you will have the chance to make the process of infusing water a family bonding activity as well. Here are other reasons for choosing homemade vitamin water over commercially made ones:

• To give a natural and delicious taste in water without the use of chemical enhancers and additives.

• It makes water look more appealing especially to kids.

• To maximize the abundance of fruits that are in season

• Contribute to the decrease in the number of waste products that harm the environment.

Chapter Three

Healthful Benefits of Homemade Vitamin Water

Now that you know that you should make your very own vitamin infused water at home, you and the rest of your family will finally have the chance to eat and, in this case, drink healthier. As a matter of fact, such type of nourishing drink provides a whole lot of benefits that you ought to know about.....

Increase Fiber In Use

Compared to taking dietary or fiber supplements, drinking vitamin water — infused with fruits and vegetables can increase the amount of fiber that your body needs to function properly. Aside from that, such drinks will help those who are not keen on eating vegetables get their needed dose of dietary fiber as well.

Fiber aids digestion, so drinking vitamin water will surely help you regulate and normalize your body's digestive processes.

Stay Hydrated

Keeping your body hydrated is a must, and it would be very difficult to accomplish if you do not like drinking plain water. I personally dislike the taste or the tastelessness of water, so infusing it made it really easy for me to hydrate and replenish all the water I have lost during the day. Remember that staying hydrated will not only keep you feeling energized, but you can also help your body distribute all the vitamins and minerals that your system needs to function. Water is also a necessary component in making sure that your internal organs are in perfect condition.

To Detoxify the Body

We are all fully aware that the body is like a sponge- it absorbs everything that it comes in contact with. For example, the air that we breathe contains pollutants that could cause harm to the body, and to be able to wash that off your system, you need to drink lots of water. And if you will be able to infuse your water with more healthy ingredients, you will have more chances of cleansing your body.

Toxins can also be found and absorbed from the food that we eat, so aside from taking on the habit of clean eating, you also need vitamin water to flush out all the unhealthy substances in the body.

Weight Loss

I have struggled with my weight since I was a child, and, believe it or not, I have tried almost every type of diet systems and diet pills just to shed the pounds. But somehow, I have failed every single of them; not only did I regain and doubled my weight, I have also developed other health problems. But when I turned to drinking vitamin water and taking on a vegan lifestyle, I have successfully managed to lose that unwanted weight, I was also able to maintain this healthier version of me. Of course, you do not have to be a vegan to achieve weight loss; but drinking vitamin water is highly recommended. Trust us, it really works!

Lowers Cholesterol and Sugar Level

Vitamin infused water will help you decrease and regulate your sugar inUse; thus helping diabetics make sure that their sugar levels are at their normal rates. And because you will not be taking in fats and empty calories, you can be sure that your cholesterol levels will no longer skyrocket.

Feeling Positive

While there are no scientific proofs with regard to this matter, you will surely start feeling positive about your life. This practice will help motivate you to really start your day right. Use your vitamin water as your encouragement to stay healthy and fit.

Encourage creativity

You will soon start experimenting on different flavor profiles that you can put together or combine to create a more vitamin loaded water. Do not be scared to try different flavors until you find the ones that you prefer to drink every day.

Lessen Food Preparation and Handling Time

One of the causes of nutrient loss is too much handling and prepping of the food that we eat. Through infusing water with fruits and vegetables, you really do not need to Use out the juicer every single day, nor do you have to cook or boil anything to smithereens. Infusing water will also allow you to bring your drinks while you are out for work, running errands or you need to go to the gym for a quick workout. You simply have to cut or slice your veggies and fruits into chunks and place them in several bottles of water, and you are good to go!

Chapter Four

Recipes

If you're a "health nut" like me you probably drink a lot of water. Unfortunately, over time you want something more interesting.

I personally use a new recipe each day – for variety.

Feel free to experiment with ingredients! Make your own recipes and feel free to share them when you write a review – I might add them in this book and give you a credit.

Tropic Paradise

Ingredients:

1/2 c. pineapple (chunks)

1 mango (cored and peeled)

1 orange (peeled and sliced)

Directions:

Add the fruit to your one quart jar.

Use your mash or wooden spoon and press the fruit so it starts to release its juices. You want to "break them" without turning them into a paste.

Now fill the jar three quarters full of ice and top off with water if you are letting it sit for night. If you want to consume within the next three to five hours fill the jar half full of ice and then top off with cold water.

Put the lid on the jar and place in the fridge for desired length of time.

Don't forget to strain!

Berry Lux

Ingredients:

1/2 lime (sliced)

1/2 orange (sliced)

1/2 lemon (sliced)

1 handful strawberries (sliced)

6 slices cucumber

Directions:

Remove the tops of the strawberries. Add the fruit to your one quart jar.

Use your mash or wooden spoon and press the fruit so it starts to release its juices. You want to "break them" without turning them into a paste.

Now fill the jar three quarters full of ice and top off with water if you are letting it sit for night. If you want to consume within the next three to five hours fill the jar half full of ice and then top off with cold water.

Put the lid on the jar and place in the fridge for desired length of time.

Don't forget to strain.

Bloody Cucumber

Ingredients:

1/2 blood orange (peeled and sliced)

1/2 cucumber (sliced)

1/2 grapefruit (peeled and sliced)

Directions:

Add the fruit to your one quart jar.

Use your mash or wooden spoon and press the fruit so it starts to release its juices. You want to "break them" without turning them into a paste.

Now fill the jar three quarters full of ice and top off with water if you are letting it sit for night. If you want to consume within the next three to five hours fill the jar half full of ice and then top off with cold water.

Put the lid on the jar and place in the fridge for desired length of time.

Don't forget to strain.

Citrusy Cantaloupe

Ingredients:

1/2 cantaloupe (orange (peeled and sliced)
1 lemon (peeled and sliced)

Directions:

Remove the rind from the cantaloupe and add the fruit to your one quart jar.

Use your mash or wooden spoon and press the fruit so it starts to release its juices. You want to "break them" without turning them into a paste.

Now fill the jar three quarters full of ice and top off with water if you are letting it sit for night. If you want to consume within the next three to five hours fill the jar half full of ice and then top off with cold water.

Put the lid on the jar and place in the fridge for desired length of time.

Don't forget to strain.

Garden light

Ingredients:

1/4 cantaloupe (cubed)

1/4 honeydew melon (cubed)

1/2 cucumber, medium (sliced)

Directions:

Remove the rind from the cantaloupe and honeydew and cut into cubes. Add the fruit to your one quart jar.

Use your mash or wooden spoon and press the fruit so it starts to release its juices. You want to "break them" without turning them into a paste.

Now fill the jar three quarters full of ice and top off with water if you are letting it sit for night. If you want to consume within the next three to five hours fill the jar half full of ice and then top off with cold water.

Blackberry Lime

Ingredients:

3 slices lime

10 blackberries

2 slices orange

Directions:

Add the fruit to your one quart jar.

Use your mash or wooden spoon and press the fruit so it starts to release its juices. You want to "break them" without turning them into a paste.

Now fill the jar three quarters full of ice and top off with water if you are letting it sit for night. If you want to consume within the next three to five hours fill the jar half full of ice and then top off with cold water.

Put the lid on the jar and place in the fridge for desired length of time.

Blue Lemon berry

Ingredients:

1 lemon slice

2 orange slices

10 blueberries

Directions:

Add the fruit to your one quart jar.

Use your mash or wooden spoon and press the fruit so it starts to release its juices. You want to "break them" without turning them into a paste.

Now fill the jar three quarters full of ice and top off with water if you are letting it sit for night. If you want to consume within the next three to five hours fill the jar half full of ice and then top off with cold water.

Put the lid on the jar and place in the fridge for desired length of time.

Don't forget to strain.

Berry Tasty Water

Ingredients:

1/2 c. raspberries

1/2 c. cherries

1/2 c. blueberries

Directions:

Remove the pits from the cherries. Add the fruit to your one quart jar.

Use your mash or wooden spoon and press the fruit so it starts to release its juices. You want to "break them" without turning them into a paste.

Now fill the jar three quarters full of ice and top off with water if you are letting it sit for night. If you want to consume within the next three to five hours fill the jar half full of ice and then top off with cold water.

Put the lid on the jar and place in the fridge for desired length of time.

Don't forget to strain.

Cherry Delight

Ingredients:

4 cubes watermelon

5 strawberries (sliced)

1/2 c. cherries

Directions:

Remove the tops of the strawberries, rind from the watermelon and pits from cherries. Add the fruit to your one quart jar.

Use your mash or wooden spoon and press the fruit so it starts to release its juices. You want to "break them" without turning them into a paste.

Now fill the jar three quarters full of ice and top off with water if you are letting it sit for night. If you want to consume within the next three to five hours fill the jar half full of ice and then top off with cold water.

Put the lid on the jar and place in the fridge for desired length of time.

Don't forget to strain.

Blue Pom Pom

Ingredients:

1/2 c. blueberries

1/2 c. raspberries

1/2 pomegranate worth of seeds

Directions:

Add the fruit to your one quart jar. You can add all the seeds from your pomegranate for a fuller flavor.

Use your mash or wooden spoon and press the fruit so it starts to release its juices. You want to "break them" without turning them into a paste.

Now fill the jar three quarters full of ice and top off with water if you are letting it sit for night. If you want to consume within the next three to five hours fill the jar half full of ice and then top off with cold water.

Put the lid on the jar and place in the fridge for desired length of time.

Don't forget to strain.

Coco-Blueberry madness

Ingredients:

1/2 c. blueberries

 1/2 quart coconut water

1/2 mandarin orange (peeled and sliced)

Directions:

Add the fruit to your one quart jar.

Use your mash or wooden spoon and press the fruit so it starts to release its juices. You want to "break them" without turning them into a paste.

Now fill the jar three quarters full of ice and top off with coconut water if you are letting it sit for night. If you want to consume within the next three to five hours fill the jar half full of ice and then top off with coconut water and the rest cold water.

You can also skip adding any water and increase the amount of coconut water depending on how strong you want the coconut flavor to be.

Put the lid on the jar and place in the fridge for desired length of time.

Don't forget to strain.

Coco-Lime Water

Ingredients:

1/2 lime (sliced)

1/2 quart coconut water

Directions:

Add the fruit to your one quart jar. Add more lime if you want a stronger flavor.

Use your mash or wooden spoon and press the lime so it starts to release its juices. You want to "break it open" without turning it into a paste.

Now fill the jar three quarters full of ice and top off with coconut water if you are letting it sit for night. If you want to consume within the next three to five hours fill the jar half full of ice and then top off with coconut water and the rest cold water.

You can also skip adding any water and increase the amount of coconut water depending on how strong you want the coconut flavor to be.

Put the lid on the jar and place in the fridge for desired length of time.

Don't forget to strain.

Raspberry Miracle

Ingredients:

1/2 c. raspberries

2 slices lemon

1/2 quart coconut water

Directions:

Add the fruit to your one quart jar.

Use your mash or wooden spoon and press the fruit so it starts to release its juices. You want to "break them" without turning them into a paste.

Now fill the jar three quarters full of ice and top off with coconut water if you are letting it sit for night. If you want to consume within the next three to five hours fill the jar half full of ice and then top off with coconut water and the rest cold water.

You can also skip adding any water and increase the amount of coconut water depending on how strong you want the coconut flavor to be.

Put the lid on the jar and place in the fridge for desired length of time.

Don't forget to strain.

Vanilla Peach

Ingredients:

2 peaches (pitted and sliced)

1 vanilla bean (sliced)

Directions:

Add fruit to your one quart jar.

Use your mash or wooden spoon and press the peaches so they start to release their juices. You want to "break them" without turning them into a paste.

Scrape out the inside of your vanilla bean and add the scrapings to the jar. You can also add the scraped vanilla bean if you want.

Now fill the jar three quarters full of ice and top off with water if you are letting it sit for night. If you want to consume within the next three to five hours fill the jar half full of ice and then top off with cold water.

Put the lid on the jar and place in the fridge for desired length of time.

Don't forget to strain.

Orange Cardamom

Ingredients:

1 tbsp. cardamom

1 vanilla bean (sliced)

1 orange, (peeled and sliced)

Directions:

Add fruit and cardamom to your one quart jar. Use your mash or wooden spoon and press everything. You want to "break them" without turning them into a paste.

Scrape out the inside of your vanilla bean and add the scrapings to the jar. You can also add the scraped vanilla bean if you want.

Now fill the jar three quarters full of ice and top off with water if you are letting it sit for night. If you want to consume within the next three to five hours fill the jar half full of ice and then top off with cold water.

Put the lid on the jar and place in the fridge for desired length of time.

Don't forget to strain.

Strawnilla

Ingredients:

11 strawberries (sliced)

1 vanilla bean (sliced lengthwise)

Directions:

Add fruit to your one quart jar.

Use your mash or wooden spoon and press the strawberries so they start to release their juices. You want to "break them" without turning them into a paste.

Scrape out the inside of your vanilla bean and add the scrapings to the jar. You can also add the scraped vanilla bean if you want.

Now fill the jar three quarters full of ice and top off with water if you are letting it sit for night. If you want to consume within the next three to five hours fill the jar half full of ice and then top off with cold water.

Put the lid on the jar and place in the fridge for desired length of time.

Don't forget to strain.

Strawberry Orange

Ingredients:

11 strawberries (sliced)

2 tea bags, chamomile tea

1 orange (sliced)

Directions:

Bring 1/2 a quart of water to a boil. Remove from heat.

Place tea bags in a separate jar, pour boiled water over them and let steep for five to ten minutes. Remove tea bags once desired strength has been achieved. Let cool.

Place your fruit into a different jar and muddle as per the usual instructions.

Pour cooled tea into jar and add ice as desired.

Place the lid on the jar and refrigerate.

Cucuapple

Ingredients:

1/2 pineapple (chunks)

 1/2 cucumber (sliced)

Directions:

Add the fruit to your one quart jar.

Use your mash or wooden spoon and press the fruit so it starts to release its juices. You want to "break them" without turning them into a paste.

Now fill the jar three quarters full of ice and top off with water if you are letting it sit for night. If you want to consume within the next three to five hours fill the jar half full of ice and then top off with cold water.

Put the lid on the jar and place in the fridge for desired length of time.

Don't forget to strain.

Orangy Lemone

Ingredients:

4 mandarin oranges

1 lemon

Directions:

Peel and cut the oranges and lemon into slices. Add the fruit to your one quart jar.

Use your mash or wooden spoon and press the fruit so it starts to release its juices. You want to "break them" without turning them into a paste.

Now fill the jar three quarters full of ice and top off with water if you are letting it sit for night. If you want to consume within the next three to five hours fill the jar half full of ice and then top off with cold water.

Put the lid on the jar and place in the fridge for desired length of time.

Don't forget to strain.

Raspberry Surprise

Ingredients:

1 lime (quartered)

11 raspberries

Directions:

Add the fruit to your one quart jar.

Use your mash or wooden spoon and press the fruit so it starts to release its juices. You want to "break them" without turning them into a paste.

Now fill the jar three quarters full of ice and top off with water if you are letting it sit for night. If you want to consume within the next three to five hours fill the jar half full of ice and then top off with cold water.

Put the lid on the jar and place in the fridge for desired length of time.

Don't forget to strain.

Pineapple Mix

Ingredients:

1 orange (sliced)

1/2 c. pineapple (cut them good)

Directions:

Add the fruit to your one quart jar.

Use your mash or wooden spoon and press the fruit so it starts to release its juices. You want to "break them" without turning them into a paste.

Now fill the jar three quarters full of ice and top off with water if you are letting it sit for night. If you want to consume within the next three to five hours fill the jar half full of ice and then top off with cold water.

Put the lid on the jar and place in the fridge for desired length of time.

Don't forget to strain.

Lemony Surprise!

Ingredients:

15 strawberries (sliced)

1 lemon (sliced)

Directions:

Use the strawberries and cut their tops off before slicing. Add the fruit to your one quart jar.

Use your mash or wooden spoon and press the fruit so it starts to release its juices. You want to "break them" without turning them into a paste.

Now fill the jar three quarters full of ice and top off with water if you are letting it sit for night. If you want to consume within the next three to five hours fill the jar half full of ice and then top off with cold water.

Put the lid on the jar and place in the fridge for desired

Starfruit Madness

Ingredients:

6 strawberries (sliced)

3 starfruit slices (peeled)

Directions:

Use the strawberries and cut their tops. Add the fruit to your one quart jar.
Use your mash or wooden spoon and press the fruit so it starts to release its juices. You want to "break them" without turning them into a paste.
Now fill the jar three quarters full of ice and top off with water if you are letting it sit for night. If you want to consume within the next three to five hours fill the jar half full of ice and then top off with cold water.
Put the lid on the jar and place in the fridge for desired length of time.
Don't forget to strain.

Pomegranate Love

Ingredients:

1/2 c. pomegranate seeds

2 lemon slices

Directions:

Add the fruit to your one quart jar.

Use your mash or wooden spoon and press the fruit so it starts to release its juices. You want to "break them" without turning them into a paste.

Now fill the jar three quarters full of ice and top off with water if you are letting it sit for night. If you want to consume within the next three to five hours fill the jar half full of ice and then top off with cold water.

Put the lid on the jar and place in the fridge for desired length of time.

Don't forget to strain.

L-Lime Delight

Ingredients:

1/2 lime (sliced)

1/2 lemon (sliced)

Directions:

Add the fruit to your one quart jar.

Use your mash or wooden spoon and press the fruit so it starts to release its juices. You want to "break them" without turning them into a paste.

Now fill the jar three quarters full of ice and top off with water if you are letting it sit for night. If you want to consume within the next three to five hours fill the jar half full of ice and then top off with cold water.

Put the lid on the jar and place in the fridge for desired length of time.

Don't forget to strain.

Ginger-Orange Madness

Ingredients:

1 piece ginger, small

1 orange (sliced)

Directions:

Use the skin off the ginger and slice into small rings. Add ginger to jar and muddle lightly. Then add the orange to your one quart jar.

Use your mash or wooden spoon and press the orange so it starts to release its juices. You want to "break it open" without turning it into a paste.

Now fill the jar three quarters full of ice and top off with water if you are letting it sit for night. If you want to consume within the next three to five hours fill the jar half full of ice and then top off with cold water.

Put the lid on the jar and place in the fridge for desired length of time.

Don't forget to strain.

Strawberry-Tangerine Water

Ingredients:

3/4 c. sliced strawberries

1 tangerine rind

Directions:

Try to avoid getting too much of the white pith from the tangerine rind. Add strawberries and rind to your one quart jar.

Use your mash or wooden spoon and press the fruit so it starts to release its juices. You want to "break them" without turning them into a paste.

Now fill the jar three quarters full of ice and top off with water if you are letting it sit for night. If you want to consume within the next three to five hours fill the jar half full of ice and then top off with cold water.

Put the lid on the jar and place in the fridge for desired length of time.

Don't forget to strain.

Blueberry Cream

Ingredients:

1/2 c. blueberries

5 raspberries

Directions:

Add the fruit to your one quart jar.

Use your mash or wooden spoon and press the fruit so it starts to release its juices. You want to "break them" without turning them into a paste.

Now fill the jar three quarters full of ice and top off with water if you are letting it sit for night. If you want to consume within the next three to five hours fill the jar half full of ice and then top off with cold water.

Put the lid on the jar and place in the fridge for desired length of time.

Don't forget to strain.

Tasty Pomegranate

Ingredients:

1/2 c. pomegranate seeds

2 oranges (peeled and sliced)

Directions:

Add the fruit to your one quart jar.

Use your mash or wooden spoon and press the fruit so it starts to release its juices. You want to "break them" without turning them into a paste.

Now fill the jar three quarters full of ice and top off with water if you are letting it sit for night. If you want to consume within the next three to five hours fill the jar half full of ice and then top off with cold water.

Put the lid on the jar and place in the fridge for desired length of time.

Don't forget to strain.

Cherry Queen

Ingredients:

10-15 cherries

1/2 lime (sliced)

Directions:

Use your mash or wooden spoon and press the fruit so it starts to release its juices. You want to "break them" without turning them into a paste.

Now fill the jar three quarters full of ice and top off with water if you are letting it sit for night. If you want to consume within the next three to five hours fill the jar half full of ice and then top off with cold water.

Put the lid on the jar and place in the fridge for desired length of time.

Don't forget to strain.

Grapefruit Apple Water

Ingredients:

1 c. pineapple (chunks)

1/2 grapefruit (sliced)

 1/2 apple (sliced)

Directions:

Add pineapple and grapefruit to your one quart jar.

Use your mash or wooden spoon and press the fruit so it starts to release its juices. You want to "break them" without turning them into a paste.

Add but do not muddle the apple and just slice thinly.

Now fill the jar three quarters full of ice and top off with water if you are letting it sit for night. If you want to consume within the next three to five hours fill the jar half full of ice and then top off with cold water.

Put the lid on the jar and place in the fridge for desired length of time.

Don't forget to strain.

Strawberry Seeds

Ingredients:

14 strawberries (tops removed and sliced)

1 c. pomegranate seeds

Directions:

Add fruit to your one quart jar.

Use your mash or wooden spoon and press the fruit so it starts to release its juices. You want to "break them" without turning them into a paste.

Now fill the jar three quarters full of ice and top off with water if you are letting it sit for night. If you want to consume within the next three to five hours fill the jar half full of ice and then top off with cold water.

Put the lid on the jar and place in the fridge for desired length of time.

Don't forget to strain.

Tropic Beauty

Ingredients:

1 c. pineapple (chunks)

1/2 c. mango (chunks

1/2 quart coconut water

Directions:

Add the fruit to your one quart jar.

Use your mash or wooden spoon and press the fruit so it starts to release its juices. You want to "break them" without turning them into a paste.

Now fill the jar three quarters full of ice and top off with coconut water if you are letting it sit for night. If you want to consume within the next three to five hours fill the jar half full of ice and then top off with coconut water and the rest cold water.

You can also skip adding any water and increase the amount of coconut water depending on how strong you want the coconut flavor to be.

Put the lid on the jar and place in the fridge for desired length of time.

Don't forget to strain.

My favorite – Maximum Alkaline

Ingredients:

4 slices cucumber

4 slices lemon (peeled, no seeds)

Directions:

Add the fruit to your one quart jar.

Use your mash or wooden spoon and press the fruit so it starts to release its juices. You want to "break them" without turning them into a paste.

Now fill the jar three quarters full of ice and top off with water if you are letting it sit for night. If you want to consume within the next three to five hours fill the jar half full of ice and then top off with cold water.

Put the lid on the jar and place in the fridge for desired length of time.

Don't forget to strain.

Blueberry Water

Ingredients:

1 diced apple (cored)

1/2 c. blueberries

Directions:

Add blueberries to your one quart jar.

Use your mash or wooden spoon and press the fruit so it starts to release its juices. You want to "break them" without turning them into a paste.

Add but do not muddle the apple and just slice thinly.

Now fill the jar three quarters full of ice and top off with water if you are letting it sit for night. If you want to consume within the next three to five hours fill the jar half full of ice and then top off with cold water.

Put the lid on the jar and place in the fridge for desired

length of time.

Don't forget to strain.

Orange Lavender

Ingredients:

1 orange (peeled and sliced)

2 lavender sprigs

Directions:

Muddle lavender sprigs and add along with the orange to your one quart jar.

Use your mash or wooden spoon and press the oranges so they start to release their juices. You want to "break them" without turning them into a paste.

Now fill the jar three quarters full of ice and top off with water if you are letting it sit for night. If you want to consume within the next three to five hours fill the jar half full of ice and then top off with cold water.

Put the lid on the jar and place in the fridge for desired length of time.

Don't forget to strain.

Minty Plum-berry

Ingredients:

4 mint leaves (chopped)

1/2 apple (sliced)

1 plum (pit removed and sliced)

Handful of blueberries

Directions:

Add mint to your one quart jar and muddle followed by your plum and blueberries.

Use your mash or wooden spoon and press the fruit so it starts to release its juices. You want to "break them" without turning them into a paste.

Add your apple but do not muddle and slice thinly for best results.

Page 67

Now fill the jar three quarters full of ice and top off with water if you are letting it sit for night. If you want to consume within the next three to five hours fill the jar half full of ice and then top off with cold water.

Put the lid on the jar and place in the fridge for desired length of time.

Don't forget to strain.

Morning honeydew

Ingredients:

3 sage leaves

5 pieces honeydew

Directions:

Use the sage leaves and tear them in half before throwing into the jar and lightly muddling them. Add the honeydew melon.

Use your mash or wooden spoon and press the honeydew melon so it starts to release its juices. You want to "break it open" without turning them into a paste.

Now fill the jar three quarters full of ice and top off with water if you are letting it sit for night. If you want to consume within the next three to five hours fill the jar half full of ice and then top off with cold water.

Page 69

Put the lid on the jar and place in the fridge for desired length of time.

Don't forget to strain.

Blackberry Leaves

Ingredients:

10-13 blackberries

10-13 raspberries

2 sage leaves

Directions:

Use the sage leaves and tear them in half before throwing them into the jar and lightly muddling them. Add the blackberries and raspberries.

Use your mash or wooden spoon and press the fruit so it starts to release its juices. You want to "break them" without turning them into a paste.

Now fill the jar three quarters full of ice and top off with water if you are letting it sit for night. If you want to consume within the next three to five hours fill the jar half full of ice and then top off with cold water.

Put the lid on the jar and place in the fridge for desired length of time.

Don't forget to strain.

Cranberry Happiness

Ingredients:

1 apple (sliced).

1/4 lemon (sliced)

1/2 cup cranberries (fresh or frozen)

1 pinch of ground nutmeg

Directions:

Add cranberries and lemon to your one quart jar.

water if you are letting it sit for night. If you want to consume within the next three to five hours fill the jar half full of ice and then top off with cold water.

Use your mash or wooden spoon and press the fruit so it starts to release its juices. You want to "break them" without turning them into a paste.

Add but do not muddle the apple and just slice thinly. Toss in the pinch of nutmeg.

Don't forget to strain.

Lavender Kiwi

Ingredients:

1/8 c. lavender

1 kiwis (peeled and sliced)

Directions:

Place lavender in the one quart jar and lightly muddle. Add in the kiwi slices.

Use your mash or wooden spoon and press the kiwi so it starts to release its juices. You want to "break it open" without turning it into a paste.

Now fill the jar three quarters full of ice and top off with water if you are letting it sit for night. If you want to consume within the next three to five hours fill the jar half full of ice and then top off with cold water.

Put the lid on the jar and place in the fridge for desired length of time.

Don't forget to strain.

Relax Lavender

Ingredients:

1/8 c. lavender

2 lemons (sliced)

Directions:

Place lavender in the one quart jar and lightly muddle. Add in the lemon slices.

Use your mash or wooden spoon and press the lemons so they start to release their juices. You want to "break them" without turning it into a paste.

Now fill the jar three quarters full of ice and top off with water if you are letting it sit for night. If you want to consume within the next three to five hours fill the jar half full of ice and then top off with cold water.

Put the lid on the jar and place in the fridge for desired length of time.

Don't forget to strain.

Cinnamon Energizer

Ingredients:

1 cinnamon stick

1/2 red apple, sliced

Directions:

Make sure to not use cinnamon powder as it will not dissolve. Add but do not muddle the apple and just slice thinly. Place the cinnamon stick in the quart jar also at this time.

Now fill the jar three quarters full of ice and top off with water if you are letting it sit for night. If you want to consume within the next three to five hours fill the jar half full of ice and then top off with cold water.

Put the lid on the jar and place in the fridge for desired length of time.

Don't forget to strain.

Pineapple Water

Ingredients:

5 thyme sprigs

1/2 c. pineapple (chunks)

Directions:

Start by tearing up the thyme sprigs and throwing them into the jar. Add pineapple to your one quart jar.

Use your mash or wooden spoon and press the pineapple so it starts to release its juices. You want to "break it open" without turning them into a paste.

Now fill the jar three quarters full of ice and top off with water if you are letting it sit for night. If you want to consume within the next three to five hours fill the jar half full of ice and then top off with cold water.

Put the lid on the jar and place in the fridge for desired length of time.

Don't forget to strain.

Fresh Leaf Orange

Ingredients:

1/2 c. cranberries

1 orange (sliced)

3 mint leaves

Directions:

Toss the mint in the one quart jar and lightly muddle.

Add the orange and cranberries next.

Use your mash or wooden spoon and press the fruit so it starts to release its juices. You want to "break them" without turning them into a paste.

Now fill the jar three quarters full of ice and top off with water if you are letting it sit for night. If you want to consume within the next three to five hours fill the jar half full of ice and then top off with cold water.

Put the lid on the jar and place in the fridge for desired length of time.

Don't forget to strain.

Strawberry leaf

Ingredients:

1 c. strawberries (tops cut off and sliced)

1/2 grapefruit (peeled and sliced)

2 sage leaves

Directions:

Use the sage leaves and tear them in half before throwing into the jar and lightly muddling them. Add the strawberries and grapefruit next.

Use your mash or wooden spoon and press the fruit so it starts to release its juices. You want to "break them" without turning them into a paste.

Now fill the jar three quarters full of ice and top off with water if you are letting it sit for night. If you want to consume within the next three to five hours fill the jar half full of ice and then top off with cold water.

Put the lid on the jar and place in the fridge for desired length of time.

Don't forget to strain.

Cucumber Rosemary

Ingredients:

2 sprigs rosemary

15 slices cucumber

1/2 grapefruit (peeled and sliced)

Directions:

Toss the rosemary sprigs into the one quart jar and lightly muddle them. Add the cucumber and grapefruit next.

Use your mash or wooden spoon and press the fruit so it starts to release its juices. You want to "break them" without turning them into a paste.

Now fill the jar three quarters full of ice and top off with water if you are letting it sit for night. If you want to consume within the next three to five hours fill the jar half full of ice and then top off with cold water.

Put the lid on the jar and place in the fridge for desired length of time.

Don't forget to strain.

Starfruit Romance

Ingredients:

3 slices orange

4 slices starfruit (cored and peeled)

2 tea bags, hibiscus

Directions:

Bring 1/2 a quart of water to a boil. Remove from heat.

Place tea bags in a separate jar, pour boiled water over them and let steep for five to ten minutes. Remove tea bags once desired strength has been achieved.

Place your fruit into a different jar and muddle as per the usual instructions after the tea has cooled down.

Pour cooled tea into jar and add ice as desired.

Place the lid on the jar and refrigerate.

Raspberry Tea Water

Ingredients:

11 raspberries

4 watermelon pieces

2 tea bags, hibiscus

Directions:

Bring 1/2 a quart of water to a boil. Remove from heat.

Place tea bags in a separate jar, pour boiled water over them and let steep for five to ten minutes. Remove tea bags once desired strength has been achieved.

Place your fruit into a different jar and muddle as per the usual instructions after the tea has cooled down.

Pour cooled tea into jar and add ice as desired.

Place the lid on the jar and refrigerate.

Hibiscus Water

Ingredients:

6 slices mandarin orange (peeled)

1/2 lime (sliced)

1 tea bag, hibiscus

Directions:

Bring 1/2 a quart of water to a boil. Remove from heat.

Place tea bags in a separate jar, pour boiled water over them and let steep for five to ten minutes. Remove tea bags once desired strength has been achieved.

Place your fruit in the jar and muddle as per the usual instructions after the tea has cooled down.

Pour cooled tea into jar and add ice as desired.

Place the lid on the jar and refrigerate.

Orange Blueberry Water

Ingredients:

11 blueberries

2 slices orange

6 basil leaves

Directions:

Use the basil leaves and tear them in half before throwing into the jar and lightly muddling them. Add the oranges and blueberries next.

Use your mash or wooden spoon and press the fruit so it starts to release its juices. You want to "break them" without turning them into a paste.

Now fill the jar three quarters full of ice and top off with water if you are letting it sit for night. If you want to consume within the next three to five hours fill the jar half full of ice and then top off with cold water.

Put the lid on the jar and place in the fridge for desired length of time.

Don't forget to strain.

Mango Water

Ingredients:

8 basil leaves

1 ripe mango (peeled and cubed)

Directions:

Use the basil leaves and tear them in half before throwing into the jar and lightly muddling them. Add the mango cubes next.

Use your mash or wooden spoon and press the mango so it starts to release its juices. You want to "break it open" without turning it into a paste.

Now fill the jar three quarters full of ice and top off with water if you are letting it sit for night. If you want to consume within the next three to five hours fill the jar half full of ice and then top off with cold water.

Put the lid on the jar and place in the fridge for desired length of time.

Don't forget to strain.

Basil Leaf Water

Ingredients:

3 basil leaves

6 strawberries (sliced)

Directions:

Use the basil leaves and tear them in half before throwing into the one quart jar and lightly muddling them. Add the strawberries next.

Use your mash or wooden spoon and press the strawberries so they start to release their juices. You want to "break them" without turning them into a paste.

Now fill the jar three quarters full of ice and top off with water if you are letting it sit for night. If you want to consume within the next three to five hours fill the jar half full of ice and then top off with cold water.

Put the lid on the jar and place in the fridge for desired length of time.

Don't forget to strain.

Watermelon Fresca

Ingredients:

5 basil leaves

1 c. cubed watermelon (no rind)

Directions:

Use the basil leaves and tear them in half before throwing into the jar and lightly muddling them. Add the watermelon cubes next.

Use your mash or wooden spoon and press the watermelon cubes so they start to release their juices. You want to "break them" without turning them into a paste.

Now fill the jar three quarters full of ice and top off with water if you are letting it sit for night. If you want to consume within the next three to five hours fill the jar half full of ice and then top off with cold water.

Put the lid on the jar and place in the fridge for desired length of time.

Don't forget to strain.

Fruit BLAST

Ingredients:

1/2 sliced orange

4 cubes watermelon

1/4 c. cherries

2 mint leaves

1/2 sliced apple

Directions:

Toss the mint leaves in the jar and lightly muddle them.

Remove the pits from the cherries and rind from the watermelon. Add cherries, watermelon and orange to the one quart jar.

Use your mash or wooden spoon and press the fruit so it starts to release its juices. You want to "break them" without turning them into a paste.

Add the apple but do not muddle and thinly slice.

Now fill the jar three quarters full of ice and top off with water if you are letting it sit for night. If you want to consume within the next three to five hours fill the jar half full of ice and then top off with cold water.

Put the lid on the jar and place in the fridge for desired length of time.

Don't forget to strain.

Healthy Mojito

Ingredients:

4 mint leaves

1 c. sliced honeydew melon

1/2 lime (sliced)

Directions:

Toss the mint leaves in the jar and lightly muddle them. Add the fruit to your one quart jar.

Use your mash or wooden spoon and press the fruit so it starts to release its juices. You want to "break them" without turning them into a paste.

Now fill the jar three quarters full of ice and top off with water if you are letting it sit for night. If you want to consume within the next three to five hours fill the jar half full of ice and then top off with cold water.

Put the lid on the jar and place in the fridge for desired length of time.

Don't forget to strain.

Mint Freshness

Ingredients:

5 mint leaves

2 oranges (peeled and sliced)

Directions:

Toss the mint leaves in the jar and lightly muddle them. Add the oranges to your one quart jar.

Use your mash or wooden spoon and press the oranges so they start to release their juices. You want to "break them" without turning them into a paste.

Now fill the jar three quarters full of ice and top off with water if you are letting it sit for night. If you want to consume within the next three to five hours fill the jar half full of ice and then top off with cold water.

Put the lid on the jar and place in the fridge for desired length of time.

Don't forget to strain.

Garden Mint

Ingredients:

3 mint leaves

1 c. cucumber (sliced)

1 dill sprig

Directions:

Toss the mint leaves and dill into the jar and lightly muddle them. Add the cucumbers to your one quart jar.

Use your mash or wooden spoon and press the cucumbers so they start to release their juices. You want to "break them" without turning them into a paste.

Now fill the jar three quarters full of ice and top off with water if you are letting it sit for night. If you want to consume within the next three to five hours fill the jar half full of ice and then top off with cold water.

Put the lid on the jar and place in the fridge for desired length of time.

Don't forget to strain.

Refreshing Mint

Ingredients:

1 mint sprig

1 c. pineapple (cut chunks)

Directions:

Toss the mint leaves in the jar and lightly muddle them. Add the pineapple chunks to your one quart jar.

Use your mash or wooden spoon and press the pineapple chunks so they start to release their juices. You want to "break them" without turning them into a paste.

Now fill the jar three quarters full of ice and top off with water if you are letting it sit for night. If you want to consume within the next three to five hours fill the jar half full of ice and then top off with cold water.

Put the lid on the jar and place in the fridge for desired length of time.

Don't forget to strain.

Straw-melon Water

Ingredients:

1/2 c. watermelon (sliced)

10 strawberries (tops cut off and sliced)

5 mint leaves

Directions:

Toss the mint leaves in the jar and lightly muddle them. Add the watermelon and strawberries to your one quart jar.

Use your mash or wooden spoon and press the watermelon and strawberries so they start to release their juices. You want to "break them" without turning them into a paste.

Now fill the jar three quarters full of ice and top off with water if you are letting it sit for night. If you want to consume within the next three to five hours fill the jar half full of ice and then top off with cold water.

Put the lid on the jar and place in the fridge for desired length of time.

Don't forget to strain.

Citrus-Lime Fresca

Ingredients:

1/2 sliced lime

1/2 sliced lemon

1/4 c. cilantro

1/2 sliced orange

Directions:

Toss the cilantro leaves in the jar and lightly muddle them. Add the citrus fruits to your one quart jar.

Use your mash or wooden spoon and press the fruit so it starts to release its juices. You want to "break them" without turning them into a paste.

Now fill the jar three quarters full of ice and top off with water if you are letting it sit for night. If you want to consume within the next three to five hours fill the jar half full of ice and then top off with cold water.

Put the lid on the jar and place in the fridge for desired length of time.

Don't forget to strain.

Melon Cubes

Ingredients:

5 cilantro leaves

4 cubes watermelon

Directions:

Tear and toss the cilantro leaves in the jar and lightly muddle them. Add the watermelon cubes to your one quart jar.

Use your mash or wooden spoon and press the watermelon cubes so they start to release their juices. You want to "break them" without turning them into a paste.

Now fill the jar three quarters full of ice and top off with water if you are letting it sit for night. If you want to consume within the next three to five hours fill the jar half full of ice and then top off with cold water.

Put the lid on the jar and place in the fridge for desired length of time.

Don't forget to strain.

Watermelon Garden

Ingredients:

5 cubes of watermelon

1/2 orange (sliced)

1 rosemary sprig

Directions:

Toss the rosemary sprig into the jar and lightly muddle. Add the watermelon and oranges to your one quart jar.

Use your mash or wooden spoon and press the fruit so it starts to release its juices. You want to "break them" without turning them into a paste.

Now fill the jar three quarters full of ice and top off with water if you are letting it sit for night. If you want to consume within the next three to five hours fill the jar half full of ice and then top off with cold water.

Put the lid on the jar and place in the fridge for desired length of time.

Don't forget to strain.

Jalapeno Spring

Ingredients:

1 sprig mint leaves

1/4 jalapeno pepper

1/2 cucumber (sliced)

Directions:

To begin this recipe, you will want to de-seed the jalapeno. To do this you will cut the top off the pepper before cutting it in half. Make sure to put on a glove and then run your thumb down the pepper's length in order to remove the pith and the seeds.

Toss the mint leaves in the jar and lightly muddle them. Add the jalapeno and cucumber to your one quart jar.

Use your mash or wooden spoon and press the jalapeno and cucumbers so they start to release their juices.

You want to "break them" without turning them into a paste.

Now fill the jar three quarters full of ice and top off with water if you are letting it sit for night. If you want to consume within the next three to five hours fill the jar half full of ice and then top off with cold water.

Put the lid on the jar and place in the fridge for desired length of time.

Don't forget to strain.

Strawberry Jalapeno

Ingredients:

11 strawberries (tops removed and sliced)
1/4 jalapeno pepper

Directions:

To begin this recipe, you will want to de-seed the jalapeno. To do this you will cut the top off the pepper before cutting it in half. Make sure to put on a glove and then run a thumb down the pepper's length in order to remove the pith and the seeds.

Toss the mint leaves in the jar and lightly muddle them. Add the jalapeno and strawberries to your one quart jar.

Use your mash or wooden spoon and press the jalapeno and strawberries so they start to release their juices. You want to "break them" without turning them into a paste.

Now fill the jar three quarters full of ice and top off with water if you are letting it sit for night. If you want to consume within the next three to five hours fill the jar half full of ice and then top off with cold water.

Put the lid on the jar and place in the fridge for desired length of time.

Don't forget to strain.

Hot Pepper Pear

Ingredients:

1/2 lemon (sliced)

1 tangerine (sliced)

1/4 c. cilantro

1/2 pear (cored and sliced)

1 hot green pepper (small, whole)

Directions:

Toss the cilantro leaves in the jar and lightly muddle them. Add the fruits and pepper to your one quart jar.

Use your mash or wooden spoon and press the fruit so it starts to release its juices. You want to "break them" without turning them into a paste.

Now fill the jar three quarters full of ice and top off with water if you are letting it sit for night. If you want to consume within the next three to five hours fill the jar half full of ice and then top off with cold water.

Put the lid on the jar and place in the fridge for desired length of time.

Don't forget to strain.

Mandarin Basil Tea

Ingredients:

2 tea bags, black tea

3 torn basil leaves

2 mandarin oranges (sliced)

Directions:

Bring 1/2 a quart of water to a boil. Remove from heat.

Place tea bags in a separate jar, pour boiled water over them and let steep for five to ten minutes. Remove tea bags once desired strength has been achieved. Let cool.

Place your basil and oranges into a different jar and muddle as per the usual instructions. Pour cooled tea into jar and add ice as desired.

Place the lid on the jar and refrigerate.

Oolong Tealicious

Ingredients:

1/2 c. cantaloupe (cubed)

2 bags, Oolong Tea

10 strawberries (tops cut off and sliced)

Directions:

Bring 1/2 a quart of water to a boil. Remove from heat.

Place tea bags in a separate jar, pour boiled water over them and let steep for five to ten minutes. Remove tea bags once desired strength has been achieved. Let cool.

Place your fruit into a different jar and muddle as per the usual instructions.

Pour cooled tea into jar and add ice as desired.

Place the lid on the jar and refrigerate.

Cinnamon Oolong

Ingredients:

1 cinnamon stick

1 orange (sliced) 2 bags, Oolong Tea

Directions:

Bring 1/2 a quart of water to a boil. Remove from heat.

Place tea bags in a separate jar, pour boiled water over them and let steep for five to ten minutes. Remove tea bags once desired strength has been achieved. Let cool.

Place your fruit into a different jar and muddle as per the usual instructions. Toss in your cinnamon stick. Pour cooled tea into jar and add ice as desired.

Place the lid on the jar and refrigerate.

Citrus Tea

Ingredients:

1/2 grapefruit (sliced and peeled)

2 tea bags, Mate tea

Directions:

Bring 1/2 a quart of water to a boil. Remove from heat.

Place tea bags in a separate jar, pour boiled water over them and let steep for five to ten minutes. Remove tea bags once desired strength has been achieved. Let cool.

Place your fruit into a different jar and muddle as per the usual instructions. Pour cooled tea into jar and add ice as desired.

Place the lid on the jar and refrigerate.

Berry Good Green Tea

Ingredients:

11 strawberries (sliced)

1 kiwi (peeled and sliced)

2 tea bags, Green tea

Directions:

Bring 1/2 a quart of water to a boil. Remove from heat.

Place tea bags in a separate jar, pour boiled water over them and let steep for five to ten minutes. Remove tea bags once desired strength has been achieved. Let cool.

Place your fruit into a different jar and muddle as per the usual instructions. Pour cooled tea into jar and add ice as desired.

Place the lid on the jar and refrigerate.

Chapter 5

Conclusion

Achieving a healthier version of yourself is not that difficult. With vitamin water, which you can make at home, you can detoxify, re-hydrate, lose weight and re-energize without the need for all those complicated processes. You can also forget about purchasing artificially made, commercial vitamin waters because going all natural is always the best way to go.

Always remember to be creative, experimental and open minded when it comes to trying out making vitamin water infusions at home. You can use the ones you find in your fridge or purchase a bunch of fruits and veggies from your local organic produce markets and try combining flavors to suit your taste Who knows, you might be able to create something that you and your entire family will keep drinking for many years!

Drinking vitamin infused water will also help you develop a better appreciation of the bounties of nature. You will learn more about the fruits and vegetables that you grew up to love and develop a better understanding of the ones that are new to you.

I really hope that this book will encourage and inspire you to Use on a healthier lifestyle.

Your Free Gift

Download my previous book on how I beat depression a few years ago.

Please visit this link for FREE Audio Version.

http://eepurl.com/bsvBc9

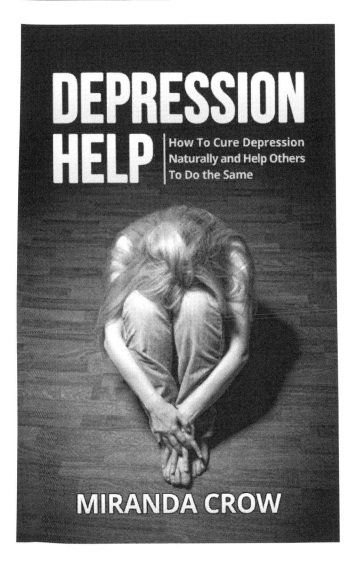

Made in the USA
San Bernardino, CA
14 May 2020

71745177R00053